Hope and Despair

Eugenio Borgna
Translated by Jamie Richards
and Adrian Nathan West

Hope and Despair

Speranza e disperazione

PETER LANG

Bruxelles · Berlin · Chennai · Lausanne · New York · Oxford

Bibliographic information published by the Deutsche Nationalbibliothek.
The German National Library lists this publication in the German National Bibliography;
detailed bibliographic data is available on the Internet at http://dnb.d-nb.de.

Library of Congress Cataloging-in-Publication Data
LCCN: 2025047197

This book has been translated thanks to a grant from the Italian Ministry of Foreign Affairs
and International Cooperation.

Questo libro è stato tradotto grazie a una sovvenzione del Ministero degli Affari Esteri e
della Cooperazione Internazionale italiano.

The translation of this work has been funded by SEPS
SEGRETARIATO EUROPEO PER LE PUBBLICAZIONI SCIENTIFICHE

S E P S
SEGRETARIATO EUROPEO PER LE PUBBLICAZIONI SCIENTIFICHE

www.seps.it - seps@seps.it

Speranza e disperazione
© 2020 Giulio Einaudi editore s.p.a., Torino

ISBN 978-3-0343-5103-4 (Print)
ISBN 978-3-0343-5101-0 (ePDF)
ISBN 978-3-0343-5102-7 (ePub)
DOI 10.3726/b23361
Dépôt légal D/2025/5678/65

© 2026 Peter Lang Group AG, Lausanne, (Switzerland)
Published by P.I.E. PETER LANG s.a., Brussels (Belgium)

info@peterlang.com

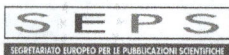

www.peterlang.com

Contents

Contents

Preface

Ilaria de Seta

As I've come to know Eugenio Borgna's publications in recent years, I was immediately struck by the grace with which he treats the dramatic themes of his work. A virtuoso of psychiatry who manages to shift mental illness not to the "normal" but to the "familiar," bridging its apparent distance without diminishing its significance in terms of patient suffering and doctors' attentiveness to care, implicitly moving the doctor-patient dyad to the center, rather than on the margins, of society.

Franco Basaglia, with his method and his law closing the asylums in Italy—oxymoronically, opening them up to end the separation and create permeability between their inmates and everyone else—enacted a revolution. Since then, many paths have been forged, in different and conflicting directions, by Basaglian converts (few, as it turns out, among his close and direct students) as well as (sometimes undeclared) and anti-Basaglia critics.

Although electroshock therapy is no longer practiced, at least for the most part, one of the lingering sticking points remains, unbelievably, the use of restraint. With the asylums closed, there are now psychiatric wards and legal procedures for involuntary commitment, from involuntary treatment to involuntary assessment, involving the use of sedatives and other practices that have been widely reported in the media, which are less violent but nonetheless a deprivation of liberty. It is notable that many writers have been "victims" of this where they could and should have simply been patients. Many psychiatric patient-writers have raised the alarm in recent years: figures like Daniele Mencarelli, Vitaliano Trevisan, Paolo Cognetti, the intellectual tips of the iceberg of a society/system adrift.

In his writings, Borgna offers his testimony as an observer who does not judge but reflects and attempts to understand, always offering a "kind" point of view on the events he recounts and the cases he describes. In the era of Medical Humanities and Narrative Medicine, Borgna represents an example of an enlightened writer who doesn't exactly decline his subjects to general interest but rather presents the "common" reader with topics that are taboo or conversely exaggerated and sensationalized by other contemporary psychiatrist writers. Borgna isn't a novelist like Tobino; he remains a doctor and researcher, but his distinctive style and the kindness permeating all his writings has drawn and appealed to readers as a pact of trust (the kind mentioned by other doctor-writers, such as the Swedish Axel Munthe and Italy's own Carlo Levi), which gives rise to loyalty, loyalty on the part of the patient but also on the part of the reader who eagerly awaits the next release. Born in Piedmont, he lived a long life, to the age of 96, and headed psychiatric wards in Pavia and then Novara, publishing some forty volumes. A glance at the titles gives non-specialists an understanding of his approach. It is a lexicon that revolves around the emotions, with nouns that form a unified semantic field—compassion, humility, hope, wisdom, harmony, solitude, silence, listening, communication, dialogue, conversation, dignity, fragility, responsibility, friendship; heart, face, eyes, spirit, sense; reason, passion, and, of course, emotion—presenting a highly innovative vision that rejects all forms of biological reductionism in a multidisciplinary perspective that puts the patient at the center.

The medical subjects covered in his vocabulary are essential (madness, melancholy, schizophrenia, anxiety, distress, depression, suicide). The few recurring adjectives offer further indication of his method (lost, wounded, unspeakable, gentle, fragile). Borgna speaks of listening, dialogue, and knowledge; he does not reject madness (the term he most often uses to refer to mental illness) but addresses it with the patient and the reader in such a way as to make it more "friendly" and less alien. This attention to words is not random; he is an eminently cultured doctor who talks about writers, and literary references and quotations are frequent. He has the merit, to his readers' benefit, of making the dramatic issues he discusses more acceptable and understandable, and of modeling respect for psychiatric patients. In 2018, he was awarded the honor of Knight Grand Cross of the Order of Merit of the Italian Republic.

I write as an editor for the publishing house that is bringing Borgna into English for the first time, with a trilogy composed of *Hope and Despair*, *Wounded Nostalgia*, and *The Madness That Is Also in Us*. Again here, one need only glance at the titles to grasp the author's aims: as a phenomenologist, opposed to any form of biological reductionism of psychiatric disorders and backed by direct clinical experience, the intention is to make madness understandable, acceptable, "normalize" it, in today's parlance, by demonstrating readers its proximity to us all. Borgna puts psychiatry into open dialogue with literature, philosophy, and the arts. The idea of publishing these meditations in English, arising from my readerly excitement at Borgna's each new publication combined with my discovery that of the great thinkers in Italy, Borgna was not at all known by the Anglophone public, was immediately welcomed by the Italian publisher Einaudi, leading to a brief but intense exchange with the author. And he expressed himself with me in the same way we find in his writing: with affection emanating from his words, bridging every distance and imparting a well-being that surprised me beyond measure. Out of respect and discretion, I would only cite the subject line of one of his emails: "ancora grazie senza fine"—endless thanks again. I would like to return this gratitude, for giving us with his wisdom and generosity an invaluable gift that we now hope to share with readers outside of Italy. These three long essays are being published under the Vectors imprint, which features short, interdisciplinary, non-specialist texts on innovative subjects to foster discussion among general educated readerships. In this case, psychiatry has a long way to go, judging by the masterly reflections of Eugenio Borgna.

Despair itself would not subsist without hope, and man would not despair if he did not hope.

— *GIACOMO LEOPARDI*, ZIBALDONE

PART I

Hope as the Endless Search for Meaning

Premise

Hope's horizons of meaning are infinite, and it isn't easy to describe or capture in all its various iterations, but first I must say that without a dialogical dimension, without an openness to the other and to the larger world of life, it is not hope. We are all swept up by whatever is happening to us in the moment, and in the illusion of not wanting to waste time, our daily lives run aground on a present devoid of past or future—of memory or hope. No one can live without hope. Giacomo Leopardi's striking words describe what perennially resurges inside us, helping us to avoid losing, or rediscover, the path to salvation, even when we are beset by anguish.

Hope is existential orientation, imagination, and destiny, disclosing a future before us that we can never predict or plan. Psychiatry, meanwhile, with its passion for categories, can't but compel us to distinguish hope from optimism, which deludes itself to orient the future according to our desires and aspirations, never recognizing their mystery. We are relation, and we have the task, the duty, of using words that don't harm the hopes of the people we come across, or with whom we have relationships of care. Words are living creatures, their content has obvious radical importance, and nonetheless, emotional tension, openness to hope, changes their meanings; hope is like a bridge that leads us out of loneliness and puts us into an endless relation with others, others who need help, or sometimes just a smile, a tear, a hello that comes from the heart. Hope is also obligation, the never-ending search for meaning, and we must learn how to capture its true and authentic value, which is entirely individual, different for each of us.

Fascinated by Hope

For a long time, since the years when I worked at the mental hospital in Novara, in the wake of listening endlessly to my patients' experiences, their sadness and angst, their confusion and despair, I've been fascinated by the subject of hope, its eclipses and its rebirths, and I've never stopped reflecting on this subject that continues to expand into ever-broader fields, not only in psychiatry, but also in other medical disciplines and areas of neuroscience. In rethinking these new developments on the subject of hope, I would note that recent books have called it a kind of medicine, claiming that illness can by defeated with words; and these trajectories, which I've followed over these many years of reflection on themes such as loneliness and silence, guilt and nostalgia, vulnerability and responsibility, happiness and sadness, despair and hope, seem to reemerge in areas that have nothing to do with psychiatry. But in addressing hope, the language of psychiatry must be radically overhauled and aligned more closely to literature and philosophy. I've written about hope in works from distant eras, but have only found a similar approach in psychiatric writings from Germany; here in Italy, they are considered utterly extraneous to the scientificity of psychiatry, not unlike other phenomenologically-oriented subjects like loneliness, kindness, affection, and nostalgia.

Generative Hope

These are some of the themes underlying the book that I wanted to write, trying to find words that will allow us to revive the hope inside each of us and make it grow, in line with Soren Kirkegaard's brilliant insight that defines hope as "passion for the possible": an opening toward a future we have yet to know, and that is born and dies with our predictions and plans, following not the rational paths of knowledge but the unpredictable ones of emotion and intuition. Hope dries up most acutely in that form of life that in psychiatry we call depression, which is nourished by deep sadness and apprehension, making it impossible to live in the future, in the yet-to-come, confining us to a fragile and precarious present constantly devoured by a past, in the absence of all transcendence. There is more than one kind of depression, and in each one, hope crumbles in different ways, and may disappear entirely.

This book aims to lay out the threads of my thinking on hope and its metamorphoses, returning to some of the considerations in my books *Expectation and Hope* and *Responsibility and Hope*. We live in an age in which we refuse to look at hope, which, in its infinite openness to the future, to the yet-to-come, change, the unexpected, the unforeseen, calls into question—at the cost of great effort and fear—what our apparently set realities are, which we get used to, sparing ourselves the effort of thinking about how to modify them and how to redeem them in a horizon of new reflections. Hope, thinking of hope, about what could happen tomorrow, doesn't leave us in peace; it keeps us away from the enchantment and certainties about the present that at least apparently have nothing to do not just with the future but also with the past. Hope is born and dies when it wants, revolutionary in its way due to its social dimension: we hope not just for ourselves, but also for others, freeing us from loneliness, the suffocating loneliness that's so painful and so prevalent today.

Hope allows us to see reality with eyes unclouded or undarkened by externalities, habits, conventions or repetitions, enabling us to open ourselves to the future and freeing us from the unrelenting prison of past and present.

Time

It's impossible to speak of hope without reflecting on time, on St. Augustine's meditations on time in the *Confessions*, which have lost none of their psychological and human significance. Allow me to cite a few lines which are special to me personally and also demonstrate the brilliance of his thought.

"For what is time? Who can easily and briefly explain it? Who can even comprehend it in thought or put the answer into words? Yet is it not true that in conversation we refer to nothing more familiarly or knowingly than time? And surely we understand it when we speak of it; we understand it also when we hear another speak of it.

"What, then, is time? If no one asks me, I know what it is. If I wish to explain it to him who asks me, I do not know. Yet I say with confidence that I know that if nothing passed away, there would be no past time; and if nothing were still coming, there would be no future time; and if there were nothing at all, there would be no present time.

"But, then, how is it that there are the two times, past and future, when even the past is now no longer and the future is now not yet? But if the present were always present, and did not pass into past time, it obviously would not be time but eternity. If, then, time present—if it be time—comes into existence only because it passes into time past, how can we say that even this is, since the cause of its being is that it will cease to be? Thus, can we not truly say that time is only as it tends toward nonbeing?"

St. Augustine, following paths that are shown to us in reading the *Confessions*, reaches his famed conclusions: "But even now it is manifest and clear that there are neither times future nor times past. Thus it is not properly said that there are three times, past, present, and future. Perhaps it might be said rightly that there are three times: a time present of things past; a time present of things present; and a time present of things future. For these three do coexist somehow in the soul, for otherwise I could not see them. The time present of things past is memory; the time present of things present is direct experience; the time present of things future is expectation. If we are allowed to speak of these things so, I see three times, and I grant that there are three. Let it still be said, then, as our misapplied custom has it: 'There are three times, past, present, and future.' I shall not be troubled by it, nor argue, nor object—always provided that what is said is understood, so that neither the future nor the past is said to exist now. There are but few things about which we speak properly—and many more about which we speak improperly—though we understand one another's meaning."

Only by starting from this inner time, this subjective time, this time of the self, which has nothing to do with clock time, the time of the hourglass, objective time, are we able to grasp the essential core of the emotions, joy and sorrow, melancholy and disquiet, hope and serenity. Inner time is the time of the soul, in which past, present and future endlessly intertwine, and in different ways in each of us; whereas clock time, chronological time, marks the passing of a time common to us all.

Hope's Existential Wellspring

Hope as an existential category cannot be understood in its emblematic radicality except in the context of philosophical reflections that allow us to approach its eidetic core: its infinite horizons of meaning. I can't help but cite the burning embers of Blaise Pascal's *Pensées* on hope and on the inner time that animates it "We scarcely ever think of the present; and if we think of it, it is only to take light from it to arrange the future. The present is never our end. The past and the present are our means; the future alone is our end. So we never live, but we hope to live; and, as we are always preparing to be happy, it is inevitable we should never be so." The dialectic and mystery of hope, the abysses of meaning contained in it, resurface from these time-defying words; and for us, for those of us who aim to practice phenomenological psychiatry, all we can do is suffuse our clinical work with the meaning contained in Pascal's reflections. We never live, but only hope to live, and so, when the high tides of despair crash over us or submerge us, is it still possible to live?

Hope Is Passion

Hope flows continuously as a leitmotif in Giacomo Leopardi's *Zibaldone*, and its pages contain dazzling images of hope that are shockingly modern. I would like to point to some that serve as foundations for my phenomenological and clinical discussion. The age in which hope and hopes fill the horizons of meaning in life is adolescence. "Before experiencing happiness—or, shall we say, what appears to be real and present happiness—we are able to feed on hopes. And if these hopes are strong and lasting, that is a time of true happiness for man, as in the period between childhood and youth. But once that happiness that I've described is lost, hopes are not enough to satisfy us, and the unhappiness of man is fixed. Apart from the fact that it is much more difficult to hope after a sad experience, in any case the vividness of experienced happiness cannot be compensated for by the lure and limited delights of hope, and man, comparing the two, always weeps over that which he has lost and which is very unlikely to return because the time of great illusions is over."

We Cannot Live Without Hope

Hopes are fragile, and easily devoured by illusions, as these other thoughts of Leopardi's tell us: "The human mind is always deceived in its hopes and always deceivable, always disappointed by hope itself and always capable of being so, not only open to but possessed by hope in the very act of ultimate desperation, the very act of suicide. Hope is like self-love, from which it is directly derived"; but we cannot live without hope: "A man without hope is absolutely incapable of living, as is one without self-love. Despair itself contains hope. Not only because a hope always remains in the depths of the heart, an idea directly or almost directly or obliquely opposed to whatever is the object of despair, but because despair itself is born from, and maintained by, the hope either to suffer less by neither hoping nor desiring anything more, and perhaps also by this means to enjoy something, or to be more free, unbound, and master of oneself and ready to do as one wants, there being nothing left to lose."

Complex considerations, and profound, which are summarized in this searing conclusion: "In short, despair itself would not subsist without hope, and man would not despair if he did not hope." Hope and despair mysteriously bleed into each other, and then, even when we are plunged into the dark evil of despair, hope may suddenly be reborn in us. "Hope, if only a spark, a drop, does not desert us, even after we have suffered the misfortune most diametrically opposed to that hope, and the most decisive." From this ensue other dazzling considerations that cannot but be read with boundless awe: "It is perhaps little or not at all or not often enough observed that hope is a passion, a way of being, so inherent and inseparable from the feeling of life, that is from life itself, like thought, and like the love of oneself, and the desire for one's own good. I live, therefore I hope, is an extremely accurate syllogism, except when we are not aware of life, as in sleep, etc."

No better definitions of the secret and mysterious elixir of hope exist than in Leopardi's gloriously arcane phenomenology.

There Is No Suicide Without Hope

Hope never dries up, not even when one chooses to die. Indeed, Leopardi says this, and I will cite his words now, though my own discussion of suicide, the consequence of a life lost to hope, will come later. "Anyone who kills himself is not really without hope, any more than he really hates himself, or does not love himself. We always have hope in each moment of our life. Each moment is a thought, and so each moment is in a way an act of desire, and an act of hope as well, an act which is always logically distinguishable from, but nonetheless in practice usually almost identical with, the act of desire, and hope is almost identical with, or certainly inseparable from, desire." Leopardi continues these considerations with his ardent desire for death, combined with fear of it. "I found myself desperately bored with life, with a very strong desire to kill myself, and had an intimation of something bad, which frightened me at the very moment that I wanted to die, and placed me immediately in a state of apprehension and anxiety"; and then the acute, lacerating perception of the discordances between the one and the other: "I have never felt so strongly the absolute conflict of the elements that form the present human condition, forced to fear for its life and to seek at all costs to preserve it, just then when it was most burdensome, and when it could resolve to be ended by its own will (but by no other cause) […] and upsets the order of things (since it encourages suicide, the thing most contrary to nature that can be imagined)."

Yet another passage shows us Leopardi's difficulty with living, and his tormented conflict between reason and passion, reason and nature. "I know full well that nature with all its might abhors suicide; I know that suicide breaches all of nature's laws more gravely than does any other human wrong-doing. But since nature was completely altered, since our life has ceased to be natural, since the happiness that nature had destined for us has fled forever and we became incurably unhappy, and since the desire for death—which according to nature we should "never even conceive of—has got us in its grip by virtue of reason and in spite of nature, why does this same reason prevent us from satisfying that desire, and from redressing in the only way possible the injuries that reason itself, and it alone, has done us?" One final consideration: "Why, after reason has fought and defeated nature in order to make us unhappy, does it then forge an alliance with nature, in order to cap our unhappiness, by preventing us from bringing it to that end which would be within our grasp?" Longing for death wells up in Leopardi from a life that has become empty of hope.

Recollections

Not the theme of suicide, but of death, and of mortally wounded hope, resurfaces in Leopardi's poetry, particularly in one of his most beautiful and unforgettable: "Recollections." Frustrated hope, wounded and bleeding nostalgia, memory, from which bright and painful images of the past come bubbling up, of death which contains them all—these are the thematic horizons of poetry. I'd like to excerpt from it a few excruciatingly beautiful stanzas.

> The wind comes, with the hour that tolls
> from the town tower. This sound, I can remember,
> was a comfort to my nights,
> when as a child I lay in my dark room
> prey to unrelenting terrors, sighing for morning.
> There's nothing here I see or feel
> but that some image doesn't live in me again,
> some sweet memory come to light.
> Sweet in itself; but knowledge of the present
> replaces it with pain, and a vain desire
> for the past, however sad, and the wish
> to say: I was. That loggia there, which faces

the day's last rays, these painted walls,
those pictured herds, and the Sun that rises
over lonely country, offered a thousand
pleasures as I lay with my omnipotent
imagination, ever eloquent and always with me.

The fourth stanza:

Hopes, hopes: O bright illusions
of my early years! Whenever I talk
I come around to you, for though time passes
and affections and ideas change,
I can't forget you. Yes, I understand
glory and honor are phantoms;
joys and things mere wishes; life produces nothing,
only senseless suffering. Yet though my years
are empty, though my mortal life
is barren and lightless, I can see
that fate is taking little from me.
Yet sometimes I think back on you, old hopes of mine,
and my sweet first imagining, and then
look at my life, so purposeless, so painful,
and see that death
is what remains for me of so much hope.
I feel my heart break, and I'm totally
inconsolable about my fate.
And when at last this death I've prayed for
is upon me and the end
of my misadventure will have come,
when earth will be an unfamiliar valley
and the future flies from view, I'm sure
I'll think of you again, and my imagining
will make me sigh again, will make me bitter
that I lived in vain, and the sweet release
of my last day will be alloyed with suffering.

The fifth stanza:

But already, in the early youthful tumult
of happiness and anguish and desire,
there were many times I prayed for death,
and sat long by that fountain there,
thinking I'd end my hope and suffering

in its waters. Later, when cruel illness
put my life in danger,
I wept for lovely youth, and for the best
of my unhappy days that died so soon.
And often, sitting late at night
on the bed that was my witness, miserably
writing poetry by my faint lantern,
I mourned my fleeting life
to the quiet night and sang myself
a song of lamentation, languishing.

The incurable wounds of the soul, the lacerations of the heart, the dizzying oscillations between frustrated hopes and hopes that spring from despair, hope against all hope, seem to me demonstrated by these verses. When death, invoked death, comes, when the valley becomes foreign territory, and when the future escapes his gaze, the poet will remember his old hopes that in spite of everything do not die drained and impalpable in his life.

(From the critical commentary on Leopardi's poem, I'd like to quote some considerations by Francesco Flora, whom I read during high school and never forgot. "'Recollections' contains the essence of all Leopardian motifs. Even in terms of scope, this is the poet's vastest lyric: it encompasses the very founts of all poetry: childhood memories, which he always regarded as poetry's deepest origins. As such, it isn't merely a poem of memories, but a song of Memory itself, the mother of all poetry"; and then: "Even the content of the poem itself is so ethereal as to seem nigh immaterial. The words are so placid and intimate they seem to be sequestered in the heart just enough for them shed the violence of newness, just enough for the most varied among them to grow accustomed to being together to form a single tender chorus. When not read aloud they seem sung if only within an aura of extreme clarity and density: they suggest not the sharp violence of the voice, but the delicateness of an echo in which all sounds are absorbed and have assumed a new sweetness." But in this poem of memory, too, the motif of hope is combined with that of his fallen youth, and of Nerina, the dead maiden).

Leopardi's poetry and prose confront us with the vertiginous oscillations of mood we find in life, helping us to look without blinders into the depths of the pain and melancholy, longing and wounded hopes we find in ourselves, and also helping us to broaden our knowledge of the human spirit in all its ambivalences and contradictions. It is true that we cannot live without hope, as Leopardi tells us in the *Zibaldone*, and an echo of this thought reemerges in his poetry, which we can't read without intense emotion every time, and which tells us how important memories are in giving fragile meaning to our lives even in their final hours.

Expectation Is Not Hope

A human experience with numerous variations, hope is a part of life, and it has a certain significance in the history of ideas, rooted in theology and philosophy, and psychiatry as well. In order to speak about hope in this book, however, I must first talk about expectation.

Expecting (or waiting) and hoping are life experiences marked by thematic consonances that are analogous but not interchangeable. There are expectations that never conclude and others that arise and resolve quickly; sometimes we endure expectations with anxiety and distress, and other times we pass through them serenely. Expectations may focus on happy occurrences, or on events that will bring pain and suffering; some expectations overlap with hope, some involve the fates of others; some expectations are renewed with each day, others continue in the same form; and there are other forms of expectation still: earthly expectations and metaphysical ones. Some are painful, some are shot through with anguish, when we fear that the future will cause all our fragile hopes to wilt.

I can't think of a better outline of the thematic consonances between psychiatry and states of expectation than the writings of Eugène Minkowski, one of the last century's great psychiatrists. His work is of seminal psycho-pathological and phenomenological importance, is deeply relevant, and possesses Bergsonian philosophical implications. This is how he defines expectation: "It englobes the whole living being, suspends his activity, and fixes him, anguished, in expectation. It contains a factor of brutal arrest and renders the individual breathless. One might say that the whole of becoming concentrated outside of the individual swoops down on him in a powerful and hostile mass, attempting to annihilate him; it is like an iceberg surging abruptly in front of the prow of a ship, which in an instant will smash fatally against it." To these considerations, which are those of a great psychiatrist who devoted his life to finding meaning to madness, and to restoring the sense of expectation and hope, Minkowski adds others equally immersed in the lush thickets of metaphor and image without which, according to his thought, psychiatry cannot address the reality and mystery of madness. "Expectation penetrates the individual to his core, fills him with terror before this unknown and unexpected mass, which will engulf him in an instant. Primary expectation is thus always connected to an intense anguish. It is always anxious expectation. This is not astonishing since it is a suspension of the activity which is life itself. Sometimes without any apparent reason the image of death, suspended in all its destructive power above us and approaching with giant steps, surges in us. Anguish and terror grip us. Powerless, we await the fatal annihilation close at hand, to which we are condemned without mercy. In the presence of an imminent danger we wait, frozen in place as if paralyzed by terror."

Expectation, in short, is not identical to hope, even as both are recognizable in one of Augustine's three dimensions of inner time: the future, the time of things to come, things that have yet to pass, and that could or could not happen.

The Expectations Inside Us

Expectation is a part of life, and I glimpsed flashes of it in the blank, wide-eyed stares, emptied and beyond hope, of patients at the Novara psychiatric hospital, faces that occasionally lacked eyes altogether. The expectation in their eyes suppressed by years of solitude and silence, sometimes dreaming, sometimes consumed by agony and resignation and despair. Their faces bore the trace of a withered, frozen adolescence, a lost and broken youth, a desiccated and drained memory. Waiting to be released, stabilized, the agony of waiting, waiting indifferently, resigned, intimidated, and depressed, fueled by patience and impatience, serene and contemplative, silent and shouted, icy and scorching, waiting as a *tending*-to (to something I know, or don't know yet), waiting as listening, nerves. Waiting for the ineffable, and as fear: as anxiety. Waiting for an illness to subside, a fever to die down. We begin each day in anticipation of things long planned, and things we would like to be new, original. We're always moving with the expectation of not being consumed by inertia and boredom, by what happens in a present that has no past and no future. Waiting is associated with moods ranging from serenity and tranquility to anxiety and dread, from apprehension to fear, from hope to despair, to the extent that there are family and social contexts capable of embracing us and listening to us. This is particularly so when the waiting is the sort that takes place in a hospital or classroom, waiting for news about a promotion or grade, and in conditions of great emotional and existential importance. It is incumbent on each of us to recognize the expectation and waiting of the people life places in our path, and to say kind and tactful words to them, filled with the hope that must save them from anguish and despair.

Hope

I would like to begin my gentle, winding journey through the boundless regions of hope starting with my own experience, particularly my experience in psychiatry, where the renewal of hope continually alternates with its eclipse. This journey will occasionally lead into areas seemingly beyond the purview of psychiatry—literature and philosophy—but which psychiatry, being not only a natural science but also a human one, and always open to listening to expectations and hopes, joy and sadness, nostalgia and every sort of spiritual unrest, all part of life, cannot disregard.

This brings me back to hope as experienced and analyzed by Eugène Minkowski. In one of his books, entitled *Lived Time*, he discusses hope. "When I hope, [...] I see the future come toward me. Hope penetrates further into the future than expectation. I do not hope for something in the present instant or in the one that immediately succeeds it but for something in the future which spreads out behind them. Freed from the embrace of the immediate future, I see, in hope, a future which is further, more ample, full of promises. And the wealth of the future now opens before my eyes." His scintillating insights continue, "But hope 'goes further' in yet another sense. It separates us from immediate contact with ambient becoming; it suppresses the embrace of expectation and permits me to look freely, far into the lived space which now opens before me. In hope, I have an intimation of all that could be in the world beyond the immediate contact which expectation achieves between becoming and the ego."

Learning about the vicissitudes of hope throughout our experiences, one of the subjects of psychiatry, is undoubtedly useful in order to sketch out and get a sense of meaning, our crises and breakdowns, in our lives. Hope draws us back into a never-ending dialogue, into a continuous relation, with the world of people and things, freeing us from the hegemony of the past and the present. Its eclipses, on the other hand, accompany the expansion of the dark nights of the soul, with their anxieties and sorrows.

Reawakening Hope

The words of those in pain, those who are immersed in sadness, melancholy, the suffering of life and finally depression, the pathological expression of these states, recuperate the semantic trajectories of hope and its castoffs, discernable by their loss of vital enthusiasm, detachment, and the emptying of their horizons, with the overwhelming expansion of the past gnawing away at their present and the desertification of their future: nothing survives of this except perhaps fragments that fail to create communication and communion with others outside ourselves. The depletion of hope in psychiatry, and not only, leads to withdrawal and dreaminess, isolation and loneliness, nostalgia for an impossible past and the ill-fated search for a beacon, any guiding light that would give life a direction. It is upon those of us who live with hope, with hopes, find ourselves before those who have lost all hope in their heart, who have been burned by anguish and despair, to bear in mind the fragility and ambivalence of our words, to be aware that we aren't always able to imbue our actions with kindness and warmth, openness and attention. Our words can be light and airy, or heavy as lead—which words do we have in our hearts when we encounter the fates, the faces and the looks, the silences and disappointments, the sadness and worry, the shyness and insecurities, the truncated hopes of those among us who are surrounded by hope's wreckage?

Clinical History

What does psychiatry have to say about hope, about a form of life apparently so far outside its purview, distant from its subjects and horizons of care? Hope in psychiatry is intertwined with melancholy, so that it is impossible to speak of one without speaking of the other. There are areas of psychiatry radically distant from the understanding of emotional content, human content, psychic suffering, melancholy, and other sensitive, careful subjects. Over the course of my career in psychiatry, during my years in the hospitals in particular, I was able to dedicate my time studying and administering care listening to pain and the silence of pain, the hoarse voice of melancholy and hope. And to illustrate this crumpled, torn form of hope, suspended and iridescent, I want to cite what one young patient of mine told me over our many hours in conversation about her melancholy and her defenseless hopes. Without her poignant human and clinical testimony, all my work on hope, including this book, would be lifeless and abstract.

The words, or some of them, of this patient, Maria Teresa, are engraved in my memory, and emerge from it luminous and whole, when I address the boundless and inexhaustible subject of hope that endures in our lives, even beyond the realm of psychiatry. "How long will I be able to endure this suffering? There are depressions that go on forever, and mine is one of them. I'm so entrenched in this pain that it seems impossible to get the pit out of my stomach. It seems impossible when I hear that I will get better. From the darkest despair to a certain serenity. You feel different from other people—I look at them and they seem like they're from another planet. I feel empty, so empty. It's like being forced to walk on broken legs. The suffering is tremendous, like searching for something you never find. From one moment to the next, you're down. I truly feel dead. I feel nothing inside, I find myself void of desire, only slightly more conscious, and as a result I feel its weight even more. I'm in an abyss."

Mornings spent in terror, as the following words make clear to us. "Yesterday morning, I began to feel unwell. This anguish returning to the surface. This sense of terror, not of fear, but of desperation. I really don't know how to keep going. I don't know what to hold onto. I realize I'm too much, but I can't hold back. Mornings spent in terror. I'm so confused, so desperate. I feel myself plummet. To bear so much, suffer this way: does that seem humane to you?" I listened to these words, all twisted together, my heart in my throat, trying with my silence to assure her of my friendly presence; but her words revealed the wrenching wounds in her soul. "I was dying yesterday morning, and time became like an eternity. Home and school make me anxious, I feel surrounded by tragedy, I feel myself going adrift, I feel empty, I don't want to live, because to live means to die. I'm trapped." These words emerge from a febrile anguish that isolated her in a stony solitude and then abated, making it possible for the patient to recall what she had gone through some days prior. "It wasn't physical suffering, but it expanded into physical distress. There was a steel vise around my heart. I felt isolated. What I remember from those days was the despair of being on the verge of tumbling into an abyss and of being unable to stop myself."

Hope in the Heart

Highs and lows: everything goes back to the way it was. "I feel terribly alone. I've got nothing to hold onto. There's nothing that gives meaning to anything. I feel desperate, if only I could cry, but I can't, I don't think I'd go so far as to kill myself, and that only deepens my suffering. If I could place my hopes in death, if I knew death was close for me, if I could choose my death, I could better bear this terrible suffering, because I'd know when it would end. I don't hope for death, though, I don't, I have no hope any more at all." The keyword of hope returns in the words of my young patient stranded in the desert of a despair that never let up. "I'm demoralized. My heart pounds as though I've just run a race. It seems practically impossible to live like this. I'm desperate. I feel again like a prisoner of anguish and despair. I live like an automaton. A month ago, there was that bright spell, now it's gone. I can't understand how it's possible to find yourself in this kind of emptiness. And the anguish, I can't shake it. The situation is overwhelming. I don't feel like myself. I'm losing my mind. I can't do this anymore." Hours and hours spent in searing emotional tension.

This anguish arose and died off endlessly, and the patient attested to the flames that burned into her soul. "I feel like a prisoner in quicksand, and my attempts to escape are becoming more and more desperate. I shout out my despair to the person closest to me: my husband. I dream of sleeping forever, really what I'm dreaming of is dying. I hate myself. It's inhumane, and I can't do it anymore, this suffering is destroying me, the thought of carrying this suffering around inside me is horrifying. It's not easy to die, and I feel myself dying."

Then things changed, and hope was reborn: a fragile and unexpected hope. "The facts leave no reason for hope. However horrible the present is, the future can only be more hopeless. I want to change, I have to hope for something. Life doesn't seem worth living." But after two months had passed, the hope that lay in the depths of the patient's words gradually transformed Maria Teresa's life.

"Yesterday, I felt a hope inside that came from nowhere, not that I was hoping for my family situation to improve, it's just that I had a hope in my heart: hope itself. At first, I thought you had to hope for something in particular, it couldn't be a general feeling without an object, but then yesterday, suddenly, a different hope was born in my heart. It was lovely, but it didn't last long. Today this hope is no longer in my heart, I've almost turned my back on this hope, which contains, actually, all sorts of things, including the future. A hope that contained the future: a hope that was life. It's not easy to put what I feel into words. The future used to scare me, I used to see it as a repetition of the present. But yesterday, I didn't feel that negativity, I didn't tell myself I had to reach this or that goal, I felt like I could believe. The future, that openness, hope opening itself, was like a new life."

These are words that show us the importance of hope, not only in illness, but in life. They are words that illuminate the shadows and focus the blurred lights better than my own, better than the words of psychiatry and perhaps even of philosophy, which are inevitably shot through with reflection rather than with the immediacy of the experience of hope. I seem to hear again in my young patient's words concerning hope the fragile traces of joy and tenderness, of kindness and nostalgia. The dark nights of the soul unexpectedly brighten, and life resumes, down paths that had seemed lost forever.

Anna

Depression takes many forms, and to demonstrate its clinical reality, I would like to accompany the story of Maria Teresa's life with that of Anna, in which there is no more future and no more hope, save after several painful and interminable months. The beautiful pages St. Augustine devotes to interior time, which is radically different from hourglass time, are recalled by the words of Anna, a young patient consumed by a sorrow very different from Maria Teresa's. Perhaps I would never have come into contact with the abysses of wounded emotions if my life in psychiatry had not brought me into contact with the many faces of spiritual pain, of the sorrow woven into it, of the longing for death, of the riven hope of the silent heart. I would have never arrived at this knowledge had I not listened long and hard, ignoring the clock, to the words of my patients at the hospital in Novara, attempting to penetrate their thoughts and their feelings, their expectations and their hopes. There was no future, there was no hope, in Anna's depression, which flared up again, radically transformed, in her body and in her relationship to others. I see her face again, her expression of unspeakable anguish, the wounds of a hope that was never regenerated by the future, despite her treatment. Let us listen to the words spoken by the depths of pain, and the dwindling of life when hope is lost: "It must be beautiful to live, but I never have. I don't feel it. Others live, I don't. I see other patients come and go, I wish I could be like them. But if I have to live like this, I'd prefer to die." The most painful experiences are those that touch on the experience of time which, in the desert of hopelessness, no longer has a future. "Time stands still, there's no more day, no more night, it's all the same. Just passing hours, but my children don't grow. I see no future, I can't, I can't see even a day ahead. Why bother building houses? Tomorrow always comes, but for me there is no tomorrow. It's tremendous, the suffering I feel. I've lost all hope. I keep trying to hope, but I just don't have hope left. I've already hoped all I can. Time doesn't move forward for me. I don't know if I'll ever see the future, I can't see it right now, it races ahead more than it ought to. I can't keep up." When she was closer to recovery, Anna said she could glimpse something of the future, and this was the first sign of a change that enabled her to be born again into hope, and bring meaning back into her life. This change in Anna, as in Maria Teresa, for that matter, is sealed by the rebirth of their smile: the luminous shadow of hope, the conclusion of all sorrow, of all maladies of the soul, and of all suffering. There is, in psychiatry, no experience more wonderful and more moving than the rebirth of a smile that adds a thread to the fleeting fabric of life: as Leopardi says, smiling and hoping are intertwined, and may undo many months of sorrow and the longing for death.

Hope's Castaways

As I have said, in the *Zibaldone*, Leopardi says there is no suicide without hope, and in some cases this is so, but far more frequently, we come to voluntary death once the hope inside us has died; and concerning suicide, I would like to quote certain thoughts of Karl Jaspers, the great psychiatrist and philosopher: "Whoever has participated up close in the drama of suicide, if they are possessed of any sense of humanity and inclined at all to look clearly into matters of the soul, will admit the need of recognizing that there is no single motive that can explain the event. In the end, it always remains a mystery." And with even greater clarity: "The simplest and most comfortable path is always to cleave to the hypothesis of mental illness. Indeed, we have gone very far along this path, to the point of declaring every suicide mentally ill. With this, the problem of the motives of suicide is resolved. The problem of suicide is hastily dispatched by placing it outside the normal world. But this is not how things are." Jaspers' considerations echo my own in psychiatry, but I would like to say further that in the genesis of suicide, the familial and social contexts have a role, at times a decisive one. And so, in life, there are seasons of fatigue, of the weariness with living, of obscure ills, and more simply of sorrow and of melancholy which, in their evolution, in their recovery, or in their trespass into suicide, are conditioned by understanding or misunderstanding, acceptance or emotional coldness in the family or sometimes in the scholastic environment, and also by the ability or inability of those tasked with tending, or curing, or listening, and building relations based on kindness and humanity, which are moreover the preconditions of the resurgence of hope, however fragile.

Yes, as Karl Jaspers says, every suicide is a mystery, and nonetheless we are called to reflect on the motivations that invariably condition its occurrence, and the importance of there being hope in its wounds, or its longing for death. The diaries, the poetry, and the letters of Cesare Pavese are a painful and cutting testimony to a life determined early on by the longing for voluntary death, which I would like to survey in its illuminating desperation. For hope cannot be fully understood unless examined in the context of a human condition that has lost or never known it, and results in suicide; and so I would like to talk about the story of Pavese's life.

The Last Illusion

The decline of hope seems to lie at the root of Cesare Pavese's suicide in Turin in August of 1950. In his letters, in his infinite letters, there is repeated talk of suicide; one in particular, from January of 1927, when he is nineteen years old, is accompanied by a poem that even today I can only read in fear and trembling, because it speaks of suicide with radical anguish and determination. There is nothing that is not despair in this poem.

I was walking one December evening
On a dark country road,
All deserted, with tumult in my heart.
I had a revolver with me.
When I was certain I was far away
From any and all persons, I aimed it at the ground
And fired.
[...]
And so, walking
Among the leafless trees, I imagined
The tremendous shock it will produce
On the night when my last illusion
And fears have abandoned me
And I will rest it against a temple
And blow out my brains.

What can we say about these painful and wrenching words that attest with apparent coldness to thoughts drifting toward the choice of voluntary death in the midst of an adolescence wounded by a precipitous despair that will never fade away? I ask myself, I have always asked myself, if this longing for death, this desert of hopelessness, was already there with Pavese in his youth and his adulthood, or whether there were, in his life, ebbs and flows that finally ended in suicide.

The above poem is accompanied by a text from October of 1927 in which the author speaks again of suicide. "Why should we take such offense at the poor suicides? You call them stupid, imbeciles, cowards, as though each of them didn't have his own terrible, immense reasons." And then: "Well, I will tell you that the suicide is a martyr, a martyr as worthy as the martyrs of any religion. And by religion, I mean any passion of the human soul, be it God or Ideas, which are just the same as gods. If a martyr is one who attests with his sufferings and his blood to the sincerity of his thoughts and his feelings in fusion, the sincerity of his no longer vulgar soul, then why must the suicide not also be a martyr, when, instead of lying (to himself, and therefore to others), of compelling himself to an effort he feels useless, to an adaptation that feels pointless and moreover foreign to him, prefers kill himself, prefers to offer himself to immense pain, to the greatest pain of all?" What Pavese says now concerning suicide lacks the disturbing incandescence and the desperate passion that springs from the poem, written a few months earlier, and yet how can one forget the dazed and mangled words with which he speaks of the person who chooses death even in the midst of an apparently happy adolescence?

The theme of suicide reemerges in two other letters sent to a friend in August of 1950, the year of Pavese's death. In one of them, he writes, "You see, when the conversation turns to you and me, my hands are tied—the differences of temperament between us are such that my own words fly back into my mouth and wound me." And further: "I think it's the music you dance to that bores into me, that makes my blood quake, that makes me scowl (but mine is the scowl of a suicide and none other). There are moments when the most banal airs grab me around the throat and I want to scream." Finally, in another letter: "But you, withered and cynical as you are, aren't at the end of your rope like me. You are young, incredibly young, you are what I was twenty-eight years ago, when I was determined to kill myself over who knows what delusion, and I didn't do it—I was curious what tomorrow would bring, curious about myself—life seemed horrible but I still found myself interesting. Now, it's the opposite: life, I know, is stupendous, but I've been cut off from it, and I did this to myself, and this is a futile tragedy, like diabetes or cancer from smoking."

The Diaries

In the diaries, in the diaries, too, which run from October 6, 1935 to August 18, 1950, a few days before his death, Pavese examines the question of suicide, which remained with him throughout his life. Did no one notice his solitude, his despair? I don't know, but again, I fear not: we live, we go on living, apparently happy, and our heart is pierced by a spiritual pain that extinguishes our hope, every hope, despite fame and its splendors. Reflecting on the life and death of Pavese, one cannot help but think of the mystery of human relations, the masks each of us wears upon our faces, in the hopes that someone will notice the pain in our smile, and the voice pleading desperately for help in silence; and at times only in a diary, or in a letter not well interpreted, do we confess. Not a few suicides, those without psychopathological antecedents, could be avoided by talking more, by being listened to more, in the family, in school, particularly in cases of young people with fragile passions and sometimes impossible hopes. I don't know—he doesn't say—whether this was the case for Pavese.

He was familiar with solitude, and in a diary entry of November 6, 1938, he writes: "I spent the whole evening sitting before a mirror to keep myself company." These words make it impossible not to glimpse in solitude the central theme of Pavese's life and death, untouched by his busy social life and his literary triumphs. The path of despair, which will lead him to suicide, gradually grows more evident, as other passages in his diary reveal. In 1936: "Only so can I explain my actual suicidal urge in life. I know that I am forever condemned to think of suicide when faced with no matter what difficulty or grief. It terrifies me. My basic principle is suicide, never committed, never to be committed, but the thought of it caresses my sensibility." And in 1938: "Why should this numb, deep-seated cheerfulness surge up through the veins and into the throat of a man who has made up his mind to kill himself? Face to face with death, nothing remains but the blunt consciousness that we are still alive."

And so, before every painful situation in life, he feels called to think of suicide without managing to explain to himself the joy that ensues; but nothing manages to give meaning to life. In 1946, suicide emerges in the diaries again: "That year, too, is finished. The hills, Turin, Rome.

You have gone through four women, published a book, written some fine poems and discovered a new form that weaves together many different threads (the dialogue of Circe). Are you happy? Yes, you are happy. You have power, you have genius, you have something to do. You are alone. Twice this year you have toyed with the idea of suicide. Everyone admires you, compliments you, dances around you. Well, then? You have never had to fight. Remember that. You never will fight. Do you count for anything with anyone?" These are thoughts of a radical, barren solitude, and we who read them, how can we not feel turmoil at the at least apparent coldness with which he speaks of suicide?

Nothing Has a Reason

In an entry from 1948, the worthlessness, the futility of life in the desert of hopelessness with desolate, disconsolate words, in the midst of searing sorrow: "When the sad evening comes and your heart is broken, for no reason, your consolation still lies in your usual thought that not even a gay, intoxicated, exalted evening has any particular reason, except perhaps a prearranged meeting, an idea that flashed across your mind that day, a trifle that might never have happened. That is, you console yourself with the thought that nothing has a reason, everything is casual. Strange. At the same time, this thought is horrifying. The fickle colors of your moods you bear in vain." Solitude is feared, but also sought as the life preserver that allows him to be free. "This need to be alone, not to feel that people ask anything of you or carry you along with them . . . ; this dread lest they should have the least right over you, and make you feel it; this obvious tactlessness by others who expect something, take you for granted in any way."

These are words that even today we read with agonizing emotion, and this returns in the entry of November 28, 1949, in which anguish is associated with harrowing experiences that seem to point at a profound psychological disturbance: "It comes at night, when I start to fall asleep. Every noise—the creaking of wood, a disturbance in the street, an unexpected far-off cry—stirs up a kind of whirlpool in my brain, a sudden, swirling whirlpool, in which my mind and the whole world are swept to ruin. In an instant I anticipate an earthquake, the end of the world. Is this a relic of the war, the air raids? Is it an acquired awareness of the possible end of the universe? It leaves me exhausted—that is the word—but what does it mean? It is not unpleasant—a light buoyant feeling, as though I had been drinking, and when I recover, my teeth are clenched. But what if, one day, I do not recover?"

These are unsettling and enigmatic testimonies to a longing for suicide that flares up with a still more febrile glow in the entries from the last year of his life.

Last Words

I would like you to listen to the painful words of despair written on March 25, 1950: "One does not kill oneself for love of a woman, but because love—any love—reveals us in our nakedness, our misery, our vulnerability, our nothingness." And yet, on May 10, there are words that seem to hint that his suicide may have been motivated by an unrequited love for Constance Dowling: "The idea is dawning on me, little by little, that, even if she does come back, it will be as though she were not here. 'I'll never forget you,' is what is said to someone one means to leave. Anyway, how did I act myself towards women who weighed me down, bored me, women I did not want?

Exactly like that. The act—the act—must not be a revenge. It must be a calm, weary renunciation, a closing of accounts, a private, rhythmic deed. The last remark."

A week later, the definitive words come. "Now, in my own way, I have gone down into the abyss: I contemplate my impotence, I feel it in my bones, and I am caught in a political responsibility that is crushing me. There is only one answer: suicide."

On August 16, he wrote to Constance Dowling: "My dear one, perhaps you are really the best—my real love. But I no longer have time to tell you so, to make you understand—and then, even if I could, there would still be the test, the test, failure. Today I see clearly that from '28 until now I have always lived under this shadow—what some would call a complex. Let them: it is something much simpler than that. And you are the spring, an elegant, incredibly sweet and lissome spring, soft, fresh, fugitive—earthy and good—'a flower from the loveliest valley of the Po,' as someone else would say. Yet, even you are only a pretext." The day afterward, the gnawing existential wounds return: "This is the first time I have drawn up a balance sheet for a year that is not yet over. In my work, then, I am king. In ten years I have done it all, if I think of the hesitations of former times [...] What have I accomplished? Nothing. For years I have ignored my shortcomings, lived as though they did not exist. I have been stoical. Was that heroism? No, I made no real effort. And then, at the first onset of this 'agonizing disquietude,' I have fallen back into the quicksand. Even since March I have struggled."

The last page of the diaries is dated 18 August: "The thing most feared in secret always happens. I write: oh Thou, have mercy. And then? All it takes is a little courage. The more the pain grows clear and definite, the more the instinct for life asserts itself and the thought of suicide recedes. It seemed easy when I thought of it. Weak women have done it. It takes humility, not pride. All this is sickening. Not words. An act. I won't write any more." On the night between August 26 and 27, he would die from an overdose of barbiturates.

We cannot live without hope, and Cesare Pavese had lost hope some time before, but from these letters and these pages in his diary there emerges an unspeakably incandescent desperation. What has managed to rouse such a radical, almost relentless protest against life without anyone suspecting its presence? The poems written a few months before his death do not display signs of this lacerating wound.

Hope as Memory of the Future

Poetry

Pavese's diaries allow us to see the motives that led him to choose death with radical determination in a desert of hopelessness—but apart from them, the poetry he wrote between March and April of 1950 attests to a passionate, burning longing for death. These are poems that arise from an emotional frenzy less ardent than what appears in his diaries and letters.

The most beautiful and famous of these is from March 22, and how can we read it today without the profoundest heartache?

> Death will come and will have your eyes—
> this death that accompanies us
> from morning till evening, unsleeping,
> deaf, like an old remorse
> or an absurd vice. Your eyes
> will be a useless word,
> a suppressed cry, a silence.
> That's what you see each morning
> when alone with yourself you lean
> toward the mirror. O precious hope,
> that day we too will know
> that you are life and you are nothingness.
>
> Death has a look for everyone.
> Death will come and will have your eyes.
> It will be like renouncing a vice,
> like seeing a dead face
> reappear in the mirror,
> like listening to a lip that's shut.
> We'll go down into the maelstrom mute.

Whose eyes will death have, accompanying us so insistently from morning to evening? Are the eyes of the beloved those that Pavese saw every morning reflected in the mirror? I don't know, but hope—the hope that he calls precious—is nothing but a painful illusion.

I would like to cite a few stanzas of another poem, "You, Wind of March," written on March 25, a work of arcane beauty and intense emotional resonance:

> You are life and death.
> In March you came
> to the naked earth—
> your shudder endures.

[…]

Now each living thing
has voice and blood.
Now earth and sky
are a strong shudder,
hope deforms them,
morning shocks them,
your step submerges them,
your breath of daybreak.
Blood of spring,
the whole earth trembles
from an ancient quake.

[…]

Hope deforms,
awaits you calls you.
You are life and death.
Your step is light.

In this poem, the sorrow of living and dying, the yearning for the beloved, is evoked in light and lulling, almost adolescent words, but words resigned, in their depths, to the fate of pain. What shall we say about these verses that speak of a hope deformed, that awaits, that calls? Was the longing for hope not entirely absent from Pavese's imagination?

No less beautiful, and no less rife with despair, is a poem of April 4 entitled "The Night You Slept." I reproduce its opening here:

Even the night resembles you,
the distant night whose tears
fall mutely in the heart's core,
and the stars pass wearied.
A cheek touches a cheek—
a cold shudder, someone
struggles and implores you, alone,
lost in you, in your fever.

Night suffers and craves the dawn,
You wretched, wincing heart.

This poem, dedicated to Constance Dowling, is shot through with vivid, nostalgic images that reflect the shadow of a yearned-for death. They are moving, wounded, tender: wearied stars, a weeping night, a wretched heart that winces.

The last poem I will cite here was written in English in April of the same year: "Last Blues, To Be Read Some Day."

Someone has died
Long time ago –
Someone who tried
But didn't know.

In this poem, in its rhythm and themes, so dark and at times impenetrable, I feel I can detect the trace of death feared and longed-for, faraway and close, imagined and yet so imminent.

Lost Hope

Pavese's suicide must not be interpreted as an expression of sorrow following the demise of his love affair with Constance Dowling, but as a choice with roots in the inner history of his life, as confirmed by the poetry he wrote at nineteen years of age, in which it is impossible not to recognize a profound spiritual unease. In short, this is not a suicide that ensued from an overwhelming, unstoppable impulse, much less the callow suicide of youth, nourished on bottomless delusions; rather, it is a suicide that followed Pavese through life like a shadow across the slipstream of hopes and ideals life did not permit him to see fulfilled. A suicide he has taken upon himself with infinitely greater resolution than the fragile and wavering sentiment of Antonia Pozzi, to whom I have devoted many pages in other writings: the hopes she harbored are not present in the diaries and letters of Pavese.

Would suicide have remained at bay if the events that marked Pavese's life had been different? The desire for suicide was already there in his adolescence, but could Constance Dowling's love have saved him from voluntary death? I don't know. I simply want to indicate the importance of the absence of hope in his life's lack of meaning. Hope is openness to a future that redeems present and past, and it is a passion for the possible that does not exclude the irruption of light even in the dark nights of the soul. Theorems, idle abstractions, illusions, these thoughts of mine that attribute such radical importance to the absence of hope in the genesis of Pavese's voluntary death—obviously, they aren't certainties, but the inner story of Pavese's life, examined in the painful traces left behind in his diaries, his letters, and his poetry, seem to me an unquestionable testimony of the abysses of pain and despair life may fall into when it knows no hope.

Toward Interiority

At this point, I ask myself, what do I feel when faced with a patient in whom I glimpse the shadow of suicide, with its sinister beguilements and its endless ambiguities? How do I avoid losing hope, and bear witness with kindness and compassion? There are patients, sunk in profound depression, walled in their autistic solitude, in the dull silence of their movements, consumed by a single idea—ending it all—who say nothing about their febrile longing for death; and sensing this state of affairs, how do I not in turn reach out desperately for words of hope? There are patients who hide their desire for death in pleasant, careless words, vague and disordered, mundane and cheerful, and how does one manage to decipher and disclose what lies beneath their apparent serenity? What hermeneutic probing, what act of listening, what words and what actions, what looks and what silences, what tears and what smiles will help to unmask this desire of theirs? And how do I control my anxiety, my angst, and make plain my own fragile hopes? How do I break through, or at least crack, the barrier of solitude in which the present is devoured by the past, and the future only serves to conjure up images of pain and suffering? How can a patient relive my words and silences, my acts and my looks, my face and my uncertainties? How do I manage to penetrate the inner life of a patient who has lost all hope and who nonetheless lives in the expectation of the fragility and splendor, the shadows and light, the distance and the closeness of the shooting star of hope?

In this book, which examines the wounds of the soul, I am attempting to offer certain fragile answers to these questions. The risk of suicide is always there in psychiatry, and this differentiates it from all other medical disciplines: differentiates it in its inalienable grasping for relations, for a rapport between doctor and patient, a reciprocity of expectations and anxieties, smiles and tears. My words attempt to give a meaning to suicide, and as a psychiatrist, in this endless dialogue with life and with death, with hope and with despair, with many patients, for example, with Francesca.

Francesca

In its deepest depths, difficult as they are to reach, psychiatry is always searching not only for a diagnosis, for a possible, fragile, ambiguous diagnosis, but also, above all, it sounds out its patients' possible longings for death. If I look back on my life in psychiatry, I cannot help but recall Francesca, my patient in these recent years, and who spoke to me about her sister's suicide and *her own* possible suicide, which, for all I knew, might have been imminent. I cannot forget the sessions that marked each week's progress: sealed by a painful, torturous silence interrupted by the odd question, prudent and hesitant, on my part, and sometimes brightened by her adolescent gaze: the adolescence of the soul. The tensions, the emotional frenzy, necessarily ran high, but Francesco never showed fatigue or apathy, impatience or indifference; was hope, perhaps, fading in her—a fragile, intermittent hope, quiet then suddenly flaring up at odd moments?

The anguish of her family, their pleas, sometimes expressed, sometimes unexpressed, the shadows that settle suddenly over the life of a patient, cutting her off, and are accompanied by other sources of pain and anguish: when to speak, when to remain silent, which mistakes and lapses to avoid, which answers to give to questions that come to a stop before the mystery of life and death? At any rate, never to surrender, never to surrender to a suicide conditioned by unfreedom and illness, by the anguish that is within us. The fate of the patient is also the doctor's fate in the final frontier of life that is suicide, and only if a community of fate is formed can a person be saved from suicide. If a patient feels that their death, the choice of a voluntary death, may in part implicate the doctor administering their cure, it will be harder for them to descend into the abyss of voluntary death. The mystery of suicide is also the mystery of a therapeutic relationship that suddenly extinguishes the desire for a voluntary death. Never forgetting the importance of the words that save us, the words that wound us, and the risk run when we respond to the questions that the patient utters, with the demand of choosing among the thousand words possible those which will do no harm: recovering a hope that has been misplaced, but is never lost, except in certain rarer forms of depression that still need words, but also medication.

Illness and Hope

I would like now to speak not of the hope that dies, not of the hope that withered in Pavese, not of the hope that remained in Maria Teresa, in Anna, and in Francesca, who did not allow themselves to be sucked into the abyss, but of the hope that must accompany doctors and anyone in general in the face of a person who is not well.

A subject that always proves troublesome is which words ought to be spoken to the person who is sick and asks for help. This is an occurrence that all of us, and not just doctors, are called to respond to one way or another: with words, with looks, with tears, with a smile, with an approach, asking permission to enter the room, greeting, a tone of voice or the act of offering a glass of water. Obvious, banal things, facile and taken for granted, and yet how important, how influential on a person's mood, on hope or its absence; and we mustn't delude ourselves into thinking the sick person cannot tell whether we ourselves have hope. These are things not easily taught, they require a personal education that seeks out and attempts to decipher the emotions and the sympathies and antipathies in particular that reside in us, about which the great German philosopher of the past century, Max Scheler, has written so extraordinarily. Yes, sympathy is of great importance (Goethe once wrote that sympathy is the premise of all knowledge) in the formation of human and social relations that possess meaning and are open to hope.

Hope, which is the intuition of what cannot be uttered, reminds us of many things. How hard it is to tell the truth without lying, for example, as the great Austrian writer Hugo von Hofmannsthal tells us; how hard it is, but how necessary, to avoid the prison of idolatry in medical prognoses, keeping in mind that there are more things in heaven and on earth than in all of our philosophy, our psychiatry, and even our most sophisticated technologies. But hope as such ought not be confused with everyday hope, with the fragile hopes that are born and die from one day to the next: hope is an inclination of the spirit that is neither naïve nor incapable of distinguishing the possible from the impossible, the curable from the incurable. Allied to that attention that Simone Weil said was a form of prayer, hope broadens the confines of the possible, it is the passion for the possible, considered not in its fragile human dimension with the cold eyes of calculating reason, but with the bright eyes of intuition and imagination, which in turn—and this is even more important—give rise to or make grow the hope that is in each of us.

Not Letting Hope Die

There is no doubt that keeping hope alive aids greatly in enduring illness. The psychological factors influencing illness are no longer deniable, but hope remains alive in us only if it is present in both the person giving and the person receiving treatment. One of the simplest, yet at the same time most important and most difficult things in life is the willingness to create human and psychological relationships with others, above all when they are ill and need help. Our own hope, which is premised on not letting others' hope die, can only grow in a contest of kindness, of compassion, those fragile and ethereal emotions and forms of life that we should seek in every moment. Here, too, hope—the experience of hope in its transcendent reality—has a social and dialogic connotation; it is never selfish, or closed in the confines of our selves, but open and radiating out into the lives of others. Hope possesses a magnetic force capable of transforming us from monads with closed windows and doors into monads with open windows and doors, of bringing light into those dark nights of the soul otherwise so difficult to escape. If hope can work these miracles, then let us view it, to quote Goethe, as a falling star that never stops falling, and illuminates our path through life.

Hope and Fear

Hope is fragile, and it can be rent and ravaged not only by indifference and despair, but also by fear. In the historic and cultural context of our time, various forms of fear are growing and spreading, stretching constantly outward and growing more painful; and fear is transforming from an individual phenomenon to a societal one. If there are multiple thematic regions of fear, what is essentially uniform is the emotional response to it: retreating into oneself, distancing oneself from relations with others and with the world of life, drowning in a solitude bordering the vortex of indifference to the values of sociality, and in the desert of lovelessness and hopelessness. You shut yourself up at home, you ask for security measures, you keep a distance from others, you submerge yourself in a frenzy of alarm, of suspicion, that causes trust and solidarity to wither, making it hard to keep alive a hope threatened by the fear of illness and of death, the fear of solitude and of difference, the fear of fragility and abandonment.

Of all the fears that are possible, quotidian and social alike, one of the most common and most frequently ignored is the fear of looking inside ourselves: the fear of following the mysterious path that leads to our inner self. Why does a fear, a fear as banal and abstract as this one, frighten us and keep us from seeing a future open to hope? Perhaps it is because we worry that there will reemerge within it the traces of a past that we absolutely do not care to recall: our weaknesses and our still-open wounds, our anguish and our sorrow, our illusions and our delusions. And the fear of hope being so fragile that life can easily wound it.

In Etty Hillesum's vibrant words: "We have to fight them daily, like fleas, those many small worries about the morrow, for they sap our energies. We make mental provision for the days to come, and everything turns out differently, quite differently. Sufficient unto the day. The things that have to be done must be done, and for the rest we must not allow ourselves to become infested with thousands of petty fears and worries, so many motions of no confidence in God… Ultimately, we have just one moral duty: to reclaim large areas of peace within ourselves, more and more peace, and to reflect it towards others. And the more peace there is in us, the more peace there will be in our troubled world." These are considerations that we should recall whenever we are overwhelmed by fear, banal fears of course, but also the fears that prevent hope from helping us along life's path so vulnerable to solitude and sorrow, to despair.

Teaching Oneself To Hope

Hope, in psychiatry, can also be understood as a bridge that leads away from loneliness and places us in an endless relationship to others, particularly with those who are suffering and need our help. In life and in psychiatry, there is a need for creative hope that can grow even in the desert of anguish and despair, amid exhaustion and the distaste for life. And here, I cannot avoid citing the dazzling words with which Ernst Bloch, the great German philosopher, begins his *Principle of Hope*, with its subtitle, *Images of a Better World*: "Who are we? Where do we come from? Where are we going? What are we waiting for? What awaits us? Many only feel confused. The ground shakes, they do not know why and with what. Theirs is a state of anxiety; if it becomes more definite, then it is fear." Later, beautifully, he exhorts us: "It is a question of learning hope. Its work does not renounce, it is in love with success rather than failure. Hope, superior to fear, is neither passive like the latter, nor locked into nothingness." And finally, "The emotion of hope goes out of itself, makes people broad instead of confining them, cannot know nearly enough of what it is that makes them inwardly aimed, of what may be allied to them outwardly. The work of this emotion requires people who throw themselves actively into what is becoming, to which they themselves belong."

These are complex words, words of extraordinary depth, that invite us never to stop learning to recognize the traces of hope in ourselves and in others and to follow them in every season of our life, seeing them as morning stars that illuminate our life path and orients us toward our destiny, which is to help others: listening to their words and grasping their silent and arcane resonances, which never cease to be born and to die. It is not easy to teach ourselves to hope, it requires wisdom, which is intuition and imagination, attention and prudence; it requires the readiness to listen to that which rises up inside us, from our interiority, and inside others as well, and a refusal to be beguiled by that which occurs in the present. Not only in the encounters that life places before us each day, but also, and above all, in encounters with patients consumed with anguish, we must understand the mysterious meaning of silent dialogue in order to intuit what these patients are feeling, what they are experiencing, what their expectations and hopes are, what shadows descend over the horizons of their lives. Those who cure must know how to keep alive the torch of hope, or at least its embers, as an inner disposition, particularly when confronted with the mode of being of psychological suffering.

Hope is the soul of that kind of psychiatry that attempts to bring to the surface the hidden resources that abide in the inner life of all of us who are ill and are seeking help. A help that can come not only from medication, necessary as it is in certain forms of psychic suffering, but also, and often more importantly, from a gentle ear and a word that comes from the heart and knows how to administer the proper dose of hope. There is not just existential hope such as Giacomo Leopardi splendidly describes it, nor is there only mystical hope, the Christian hope we read of in the wonderful letters of St. Paul; there is also hope as transcendence, as opening ourselves to others, as attunement to the infinite; and it is hope that allows us to live.

Hope is the Memory of the Future

Memory is born from the past and lives from the past; hope lives from the future and is directed toward the future; and yet, these two ways of experiencing time are not radically distinct. Memories are continually reborn from the past, like an albatross taking flight and soaring from one mood to the other, and in this way, influence our manner of looking at the future. Hopes are, at least in part, nourished by things we have experienced, or that are tucked away in our memory, and in this way our memories are reflected in the hopes that abide inside us. In this flow back and forth of lived experiences from past to present, and present to future, from memory to vision, and from vision to expectation, there is an infinite circularity that advances from memory to hope, and from hope to memory. Rooted in this circularity of experience is that beautiful image of Gabriel Marcel's that defines hope as the memory of the future: the same thing St. Augustine affirms in different words in his *Confessions*. I would like to excerpt a few passages here that lead one to reflect specifically on the possible relations between hope and memory, which is the source of all possible images.

"Some things appear immediately, but others require to be searched for longer, and then dragged out, as it were, from some hidden recess. Other things hurry forth in crowds, on the other hand, and while something else is sought and inquired for, they leap into view as if to say, 'Is it not we, perhaps?' These I brush away with the hand of my heart from the face of my memory, until finally the thing I want makes its appearance out of its secret cell. Some things suggest themselves without effort, and in continuous order, just as they are called for—the things that come first give place to those that follow, and in so doing are treasured up again to be forthcoming when I want them." Memories have a face, a face that transforms into thousands of other faces, when our emotions change; and the eyes of the soul look more luminously than those eyes that are the mere organs of sight.

Psychiatry cannot dispense with other intuitions of St. Augustine's that help us to better understand how memory generates images of hope. "All this I do within myself, in that huge hall of my memory. For in it, heaven, earth, and sea are present to me, and whatever I can cogitate about them—except what I have forgotten. There also I meet myself and recall myself—what, when, or where I did a thing, and how I felt when I did it. There are all the things that I remember, either having experienced them myself or been told about them by others. Out of the same storehouse, with these past impressions, I can construct now this, now that, image of things that I either have experienced or have believed on the basis of experience—and from these I can further construct future actions, events, and hopes; and I can meditate on all these things as if they were present. "I will do this or that"—I say to myself in that vast recess of my mind, with its full store of so many and such great images—"and this or that will follow upon it." "O that this or that could happen!" "God prevent this or that." I speak to myself in this way; and when I speak, the images of what I am speaking about are present out of the same store of memory; and if the images were absent I could say nothing at all about them."

St. Augustine's words tell us with startling modernity how experiences lived in the past interweave with those we will live in the future in a continuous circularity, salvaging from the past the things that we wished to do and haven't done and that we might still yet do, in the wake of a creative longing which one may experience only if one is accustomed to diving into oneself, into those inner regions of our dispositions and hopes, our anxieties and the turmoil in our souls. It isn't easy, I repeat, because we are always frightened of discovering ways of being and living which we thought were foreign to our own lives.

Communion as the Root of Hope

In a film of sparkling lyrical grace, Ingmar Bergman's *Wild Strawberries*—to take a different thematic angle—despair and hope are intertwined, and I would like to say something about each. In despair, in this human condition that wanders so far away from hope, one lives in such a way that time never passes, and for this reason, despair can be defined as the consciousness of closed time: of time as a prison. That is, in despair, one lives in an interior, subjective time, with no future, with nothing to await, confined to the past and the present. Beyond the linear dimension of time, the time of the clock and the hourglass, there is the inner dimension, the dimension of the self, which St. Augustine has analyzed so admirably in his *Confessions*, and which is composed of the past, the present, and the future, all intertwined. In the dream of the film's protagonist, Isak Borg, the stoppage of time, the end of time, the sign of irrevocable death, is expressed in the image of the clock without hands outside a store, and in Isak Borg's own pocket watch. Despair makes us lose time, it makes us lose the world, immersing us in that anguish of death lived in terms of its fatal imminence. In the dream are reflected the painful shadows of the human condition lost in the desert of hopelessness: the despair that forms part of life, and from which, as Giacomo Leopardi tells us in the *Zibaldone*, the figure of hope can enigmatically rise again, just as the film shows.

On the journey—a metaphor for life—that the film's protagonist undertakes from Stockholm to the university town of Lund, where Isak Borg has taught for many years, there occur dreams and encounters that attest to an inexpressible rebirth of hope. *Wild Strawberries* is also a film of memory and hope, and there are no memories and hopes without time, inner time, the time of the self. The radiant images of the past, which seal the final dream of the protagonist, are possible because hope has been reborn in his life. His memory is immersed in time, is born from the past and lives from the past; and from lived memory, emotional memory, involuntary memory, which is not calculating memory, there emerge once more those memories that weave together endlessly with our individual ways of hoping. Hope feeds also on our life experiences, which are hidden, almost imprisoned, in memory, and in this sense, memories mirror one another—let me repeat—in the hopes that remain within us: in the uninterrupted resurgence of experiences which cross the border from the past to the present, from the present to the future, from memory to intuition, and from intuition to expectation. The swarms of images and reminiscences that rise up from memory, reborn from the deepest, most secret places of the soul, along with Isak Borg's encounters that day, have helped submerge his life, what is left of his life, in the springs of hope, which shine very brightly in a final dream in which he returns in memory to the happy days of his adolescence, and above all, to his beloved cousin Sara at the vacation home and the strawberry patch, but also at the lakeshore, where he finds again his mother and father lying on the grass, dressed in white, waving.

Waking from his dream, in which, at last, he smiles, his life is flooded with a hope for everything unexpected that transforms his way of living, of living with his son and his daughter-in-law, pointing to the not-taken path that leads him to the rediscovery of the meaning of life: the path of communion with hope. Without hope, the present and the past cannot emerge from the prison of the momentary, of the instant, of the occasional, of the ephemeral. *Hopes* are not *hope*, *l'espoir* is not *l'espérance*, is not what Charles Péguy calls *la petite fille Espérance*; and hope, the hope that Bergman's beautiful film brings to our minds, is fragile and friable, vulnerable to the banality of evil, and yet, without it, it is impossible to grasp the meaning of life. These are things that lead me back to the sprightly but profound words of Gabriel Marcel: he who hopes says not only "I hope" but also "I place my hope in you" and "I hope for us." And this is because hoping is trusting in a being that can be called *you*. Hope, then, is necessarily communion: "I hope in you for us." And the life of Isak Borg attests to this splendid intuition, this story of a life drowning in suffering and loneliness, and saved by that hope which is dialogue and communion.

The Duty of Hope

If hope lacks a dialogic dimension, open to others and to the unexpected, it isn't hope: just as psychiatry is either social or is not psychiatry at all. If hope is inside us, what happenes in the relations between two people is always something new: our life opens itself to the possible that is concealed within the impossible, to the utterable sealed within the unutterable. Without hoping for others, too, hope is reduced to one of many other emotions that are born and die. We are all fascinated by what is taking place now, at the present moment, and in the illusion of not wasting time our present founders on the rocks of a present that has neither memory nor hope. Plans and projects pile up, but they fail to account for the unforeseen and unexpected. Hope distances us from the present, is rooted and embodied in the pulsating material of our lives, nourished by memory: not just on the future, but on the memory of the future.

Hope throws open before us a vision of the future open to many possible influences from life. This is the source of its beauty. Hope, which trusts in the future, without knowing what it holds, must not be confused with optimism, which does not know the mystery of the future.

Words are living creatures, especially when we are confronted with matters of such importance as expectation and hope, illusion and disillusion, anguish and despair, the last of which, in its most extreme form, leads to an inexorable longing for death, for voluntary death. Words change with the changing of moods, and it is not always necessary to speak them, they can be suppressed and we can communicate with the eyes, with a smile, with a tear, with a caress.

The eyes are essential to the formation of human relations based on kindness and compassion, on mercy and solidarity. Looking a person in the eyes is itself listening and being listened to, and we should never forget this, not only in psychiatry, but in our infinite encounters with others in life. We have the moral obligation to prevent hope from dying within ourselves so that we may allow it to be born again in those who have lost it, and in this sense, hope possesses a revolutionary value: it disturbs us, it does not hold us prisoner in negligible habits and conventions, it frees us from prejudices that refuse to grasp reality in its spontaneity and human richness and that in this way cause our lives to wither.

Hope as Indescribable Human Experience

Hope as transcendence, as emotion, mood, sentiment, virtue, as an indescribable human experience, takes us beyond pain and anguish, silence and madness, so that we grasp and recover meaning: the powerful common thread of an alterity that breaks through the confines of our selves, of our monadic solitude. Perhaps it is easier to define hope moving from the experience of despair, in which time stops and is frozen in a present that borders on the past but has no foothold in the future. In despair, as Pavese's diaries and poems show us, meaning, ultimate meaning, resides only in dying and death, whereas hope entails unceasing movement into the future. Some of us, by hoping, are carriers of hope for others, and the radiant light of hope brightens the shadows, the dark nights of St. John of the Cross, reviving a delicate rainbow: a shimmering ray of dialogue and communication. Hope brings life back into faces, eyes, and tears, and prayer in turn is the source of unexpected and mysterious hopes: as in Mother Teresa and Anna Maria

Canopi (founder of the Benedictine community of San Giulio amid the stunning beauty of Lake Orta), as in Blanche de la Force and Constance of Saint-Denis, the two Carmelites of the Monastery of Compiègne rendered immortal by the incomparable visionary creativity of Georges Bernanos.

The hope I write about in the wake of my therapeutic experiences at the women's psychiatric hospital in Novara is the hope that survives the erosion of all quotidian hopes, the hope that, despite everything, helps us to bear sadness and *taedium vitae*, melancholy and ennui, and is reborn endlessly even in the arms of despair. What is this hope, so secret and so elusive, so arcane and so mysterious, and yet palpable and almost tangible, that saves us even when illness and pain descend upon us and imprison us in a life that grows arid, even into a desert? It is a hope that searches not for the iridescent butterflies of illusions and appearances, but is the insight that life can contain the unexpected and incalculable, the unforeseeable and thus unhoped for.

The Massacre of Human Hope

The confines of hope are vast, unspeakably so, even if we tend to look to our own hopes, and not to those of others distant from us—or rather, those whom we see as distant—even as their lives are fatefully intertwined with ours in human, utterly human affairs that should join us in solidarity and commonality of intent. And I would be remiss not to say something here about what is happening in the Mediterranean, lined with ships carrying to safer shores children and young adults and elderly people who are fleeing death, fleeing abominable living conditions, seeking a free and dignified life not ravaged by indifference and violence. We see their faces, the unspeakable suffering in their eyes, begging for a simple gesture of human and Christian solidarity, and we are incapable of giving it, or even consciously unwilling to give it. They are not our responsibility, and yet, how frightful our measure of indifference, I fear, compared to the dashed expectations and hopes of those people we see on our televisions and in the streets of our cities, when we forget the inalienable ethical value of solidarity.

Their thoughts, their expectations and hopes, their desires and dreams, their desperate resignation to fate aren't so hard to imagine, and yet I wonder how it is possible to be indifferent to their infinite suffering and infinite loneliness, their unexpressed cry for help. There is no hope, no solidarity, no attention paid to the wounds in their bodies and souls. These heartrending images, flashing one past the other on television, what indignant and bitter emotional resonances have they awakened in our hearts frozen by indifference, resignation, and forgetfulness? It is painful to contemplate the wounded hopes that push people young and not so young from their inhospitable lands only to be cruelly decimated.

The massacre of human hope is one of the most painful things we are witnessing today, and if it makes any sense at all to write yet another book on hope, on expectation and hope, it is to reflect at length upon hope's abandonment, the human and social consequences of the loss and abrogation of hope, which are now more urgent than any abstract discourse about the philosophy or the sociology of hope. Psychiatry brings us closer to not-infrequently hidden aspects of hope, to those in particular which relate to interiority, that path that leads to the abysses of interiority within us to which psychological suffering may provide the clearest access. Hope, as psychiatry can still tell us, helps us to reconceive loneliness and painful longing, guilt and indifference, the silence of the heart and the inability to love, apathy and aggressivity, selfishness and coldness, which are always present in the realm of life.

Hope's Healing Power

What were my hopes in life, and how can I describe them? I can only point to certain sensitive threads that have followed me in my life as a psychiatrist, above all in my contact with patients past and present whom I've tried to help in the hope that my words have done them good, and have been heard with the meaning I hoped to give them. I'm not sure whether this is what actually happened, and for that matter, woe to those psychiatrists trafficking in certainties: there is no certainty in psychiatry, only hope, expectations, for words to mitigate patients' anguish, to broaden the horizons of a hope that is not permanently imprisoned by plans and appearances.

Words in psychiatry, my words, need hope more than ever, a hope that transcends the confines of the rational and the real, when I find patients in whom I glimpse or intuit the yearning for, the fascination with, suicide. One wrong word, one out-of-place smile or tear, and all hope is erased. I have no certainties, as I said, and I never could: reason is always defeated by the emotions of the person giving treatment and the person receiving it, who are continually modifying one another's perceptions. And yet, if we don't give space to hope, healing words will never be found, because only openness to a future in which the unexpected and unhoped-for can occur can allow us to be the mediating forces of salvation. All the hopes I've had in my life, all the hopes that have been dashed by reality—hopes without which I never have been able to find the right words or even to keep hope alive in those I was treating.

How do we sustain, or conserve, hope in ourselves when we are submerged in pain or illness, loneliness or the loss of a loved one? How do we attest to hope, the fruits of our hopes, the fruits of our sufferings; how do we tell another person the words, how do we do the things that can make hope grow again in their barren hearts? What is the significance of method, qualifications, technical knowledge in extreme situations that are a question of life and death? Words, always at risk of wounding, of amplifying another's despair, and the actions that may mitigate it: squeezing a hand, smiling, stopping the flow of tears without denying their meaning, and then looking a person in the eye, seeing one's own reflection and one's own eyes in the eyes of others, in the *you* that stands before me. Simply hoping is one of life's beautiful things, but still more beautiful is to feed the hopes of the other with our words, with our eyes, marrying the language of words with the language of the living body and its horizons of meaning, which may be essential in saving a life where hope has been lost. A word, a look, a caress, a sigh, suddenly tear through the darkness, striking down the fence posts of fear and anguish, disquiet and loneliness, timidity and reserve, in the gleaming dawn and light of a new day and a new hope. These are the magical moments in life, unexpected and unexplored, a hand squeezing another in silence, hope flourishing fragile and luminous, changing our way of looking at the world, amplifying the compassion and kindness in our hearts.

Bonds

The phenomenological categories of hope and of religion overlap and diverge, interweave and reflect each other. Christian hope has God as the infinite wellspring of relations, human hope has the Other, which suffers and asks for help and is loved as a *you*, in a horizon of trust. The anguish of living and dying is not irrelevant to the subject, to the presence or absence, of hope. Again, when words try to define and explain the sphere of the unspeakable and the ineffable, they grow so weak and so precarious, so ethereal and so ungraspable, that they lose their consistency. Perhaps it is anguish that cannot do without hope, to which the future presents itself in radically different ways.

Hope as a horizon open to the possible, to the passion for the possible, in the Kierkegaardian sense that draws on one of its essential aspects that we should always look to, because it is simple and concrete, incisive, ethically and semantically sweeping, not at all conventional, and even less ideological. In saying this, I cannot but add that the closure of the mental asylums in Italy, an inconceivable revolution, and the shift to psychiatric hospitals and outpatient care, would not have been possible had Franco Basaglia not possessed a hope that was a passion for the possible and repealed the centuries-old way of doing psychology based on the conviction that madness was simple aggressivity and violence that demanded enclosure, walls, segregation, closed doors and windows, high doses of medication and rampant use of restraints. Every change in this way of doing things had been considered scientifically impossible, and yet, as violence and restraint were banished, in one of the two asylums in Novara, the one I oversaw, there was a recovery of the dignity and sensibility of those people that the psychiatry of the time had failed to see. Hope animated our working group, our doctors, our nuns, and our nurses, and hope was reborn within our asylum, even if in ways that can't be compared with what Basaglia was doing in Trieste. Was madness not defined by Clemens Brentano, the great German Romantic poet, as the unhappy sister of poetry? True, this unhappiness may be anguish, may be the longing for voluntary death, may be melancholy, may be the loss of all possible happiness, but it is also a sensibility and dignity that cannot be revoked.

Ethics of Hope

In an essay on Goethe's *Elective Affinities*, Walter Benjamin's discussion of hope expands its semantic confines and recalls to us Edoardo and Ottilie, the two lovers who are protagonists of the novel. "For in the symbol of the star, the hope that Goethe had to conceive for the lovers had once appeared to him. That sentence, which to speak with Holderlin contains the caesura of the work and in which, while the embracing lovers seal their fate, everything pauses, reads: 'Hope shot across the sky above their heads like a falling star.' They are unaware of it, of course, and it could not be said any more clearly that the last hope is never such to him who cherishes it but is the last only to those for whom it is cherished." Goethe's brilliant image tells us that hope, a falling star, cannot as easily be seen if our eyes are not bathed in tears.

Benjamin's essay closes with words whose burning ethical significance we should never forget, not only in psychology, but in life as well: "Only for the sake of the hopeless have we been given hope." If hope does not abide in the heart of the person treating or attending to another who is ill, then the all-consuming flame of pain and despair, the bleeding wounds of the soul, will never vanish. Hope arises again within us and expands the bounds of care, and hope is the antidote to the melancholy so tightly linked to psychic suffering, to the loneliness that is its painful and bitter consequence. To try and stem anguish and fear, uncertainty and despair, voluntary death, is the task of every psychiatrist who, with his infinite masks, feels the need to orient himself toward the future, the most fragile and most obstinate of the basic structures of our lives.

Hope, then, is not simply the pretext for the understanding of that which occurs in the forms of life sealed by pain; it is also the premise of healing in the sense that, if hope does not live in the healer's heart, then all therapeutic strategies are significantly weakened. Only if there is in us a drop, a scintilla of hope, will we have the necessary patience to listen to and interpret the words and the silences of patients consumed by anguish and perhaps by the longing for death.

Final Questions

I would like to ask what our habits are when we analyze our thoughts and our emotions and immerse ourselves in those of others. We should never forget that the stance we take inwardly, our ideas about illness, about psychiatric illness in particular, our inapposite words, make suffering and despair grow in the hearts of the ill and well alike; how, then, can we not be responsible with our words, or with our actions, distressed, frightened, discouraged, or indifferent? Not to let die within us the hope for a psychiatric cure means to keep present the inner resources that every patient possesses, and to trust in them, beyond all diagnoses and protocols. I would like to ask further to what extent the person who teaches must feel responsible for the presence or absence of hope in his pupils. Would a school in which the teacher creates a climate impregnated with hope not manage to reawaken it even in the most timid students, those emotionally lost in anguish and sorrow, in turmoil and despair? If hope is part of the instructor's way of being, would dialogue not be less asymmetrical than otherwise? Among instructors, would those with the greatest capacity to attest to hope within themselves not be those best inclined to listen and understand the silent cry for help among the most fragile and insecure students? If an instructor is incapable of recognizing hope in a young person, timid, perhaps, consumed by anxiety and insecurity, he cannot help him in school or in life. In school today, and not only in families, the subject of hope, of knowing how to look not only at the present but also at the past, at memory, and at the future, at hope, is increasingly important.

Hoping Against All Hope

I wouldn't want to approach the conclusion of my words here without evoking certain passages of St. Paul's Epistle to the Romans that speak of hope. He defines it thus (8:24-25): "For we are saved by hope: but hope that is seen is not hope: for what a man seeth, why doth he yet hope for? But if we hope for that we see not, then do we with patience wait for it." Elsewhere, St. Paul inscribes hope in a radically theological context (5:1-6): "Therefore being justified by faith, we have peace with God through our Lord Jesus Christ: By whom also we have access by faith into this grace wherein we stand, and rejoice in hope of the glory of God. And not only so, but we glory in tribulations also: knowing that tribulation worketh patience; And patience, experience; and experience, hope: And hope maketh not ashamed; because the love of God is shed abroad in our hearts by the Holy Ghost which is given unto us. For when we were yet without strength, in due time Christ died for the ungodly." And in Hebrews: "Now faith is the substance of things hoped for, the evidence of things not seen."

These are well-known words, but at times it's necessary to reread them; they open forgotten or unknown horizons of life, about which Karl Barth has written things of dizzying profundity. True, the Christian's faith does not crack even when human hope dies, and the words of Saint Paul are the ineffable testimony thereto.

Flashback

My path in search of hope, that falling star that passes before us, leaving a mysterious ray of light behind, is nearly at an end. How might I summarize the considerations it has led me to? Hope is part of life, and it isn't easy, or perhaps even possible, to live without hope, which allows us to see reality with eyes not clouded by the superficial, the conventional, and aids us in opening ourselves to the future without remaining prisoner to that which occurred in the past and that which is occurring in the present. I have found hope, the birth and death of hope, in psychiatry, listening to patients in the places where I've worked, and in this book I have described the experiences of young patients in whom hope was interwoven with loss and loss in turn with the rebirth of hope, with each encroaching on the other and each demanding to be understood in its reciprocal relationship with the other. This has led me to lay out certain notions concerning suicide, which is the extreme expression of a life from which every spark of hope has retreated. From Cesare Pavese's letters, diaries, and poems I have excerpted fragments from that path that led him to the desire for a voluntary death even when he was still an adolescent. As Leopardi, who sensed its attraction in his youth, recognized, voluntary death is linked to the recession of hope; and to proceed in my thinking required that I ask myself how it is possible to lose hope, and how one can attest to the loss of hope in clinical interviews with patients consumed by the longing for voluntary death.

Hope is fragile, we are frightened of losing it, and I have not managed to avoid talking about the fears that overwhelm us today and that make it difficult to keep hope alive and to exhibit. It is true, hope lives on the future, but it also lives on the past; and again, with St. Augustine, hope as the memory of the future is interwoven with experiences from childhood and adolescence and moments of dialogue and communion; and our duty is to practice that hope which cannot be confused with optimism.

The final stretch of my comments focuses on other connotations of hope: its openness to a communal view of life, the duty to entrust ourselves to a hope that we do not let die in us (and here, a dazzling fragment by Heraclitus: "If you do not hope for the unexpected, you will not find it: for there is no path nor search that leads to it"), never forgetting its ethical foundations and its human and social dimension, open to the understanding of pain and anguish, sorrow, the weariness of living, and not ignoring its overlap with the Christian justification of hope that the Pauline epistles present to us.

Conclusion

I would like to conclude by quoting an unsettling thought from Franz Kafka that takes us to the edge of the abyss. "Man cannot live without a permanent trust in something indestructible in himself, though both the indestructible element and the trust may remain permanently hidden from him. One of the ways in which this hiddenness can express itself is through faith in a personal god."

With this, my book comes to a close: a book on hope, on the metamorphoses and eclipses we may come across in the course of our lives, perhaps without recognizing them, consumed as we are by carelessness and indifference, by apathy and boredom, by selfishness and the silence of the heart. My wish is that these pages should engender an invitation to rethink the values of kindness and compassion, of welcoming and listening, which are the premise of a life that rediscovers and comes to know the fragile and audacious horizons of hope without which it is impossible to live with dignity, as, I repeat again, Giacomo Leopardi has written in those pages of his *Zibaldone* that we should never cease to read and meditate upon.

Bibliography

Augustine. *The Confessions of St. Augustine*. Translated by Albert C. Outler.

Barth, Karl. *The Epistle to the Romans*. Translated by Edwyn C. Hoskyns. Oxford University Press: 1968.

Benjamin, Walter. *Selected Writings Volume 1: 1913-1926*. Michael W. Jennings, ed. Harvard University Press, 1996.

Bernanos, Georges. *The Carmelites*. Translated by Gerard Hopkins. Fontana: 1961.

Binswanger, Ludwig. *Schizophrenie*. Neske: 1957.

Bloch, Ernst. *The Principle of Hope*. Translated by Neville Plaice, Stephen Plaice, and Paul Knight. The MIT Press, 1986.

Borgna, Eugenio, *La malinconia come metamorfosi della speranza*, in "Rivista sperimentale di Freniatria," CI (1977), pp. 7-39.

Malinconia. Feltrinelli: 1992.

L'attesa e la Speranza. Feltrinelli: 2005.

L'attesa le attese, in "Note di pastorale giovanile," September 2014.

L'ascolto gentile. Einaudi, Torino 2017.

Le parole che ci salvano (taken from the volumes *La fragilità che è in noi* and *Parlarsi e Responsabilità e speranza*). Einaudi: 2017.

La nostalgia ferita. Einaudi: 2018.

Il fiume della vita. Feltrinelli: 2020.

Heraclitus. *Fragments*. Translated by Bruce Haxton. Penguin: 2003.

John of the Cross. *Collected Works*. Translated by Kieran Kanavaugh et al. ICS Publications: 1991.

Goethe, Johann Wolfgang von. *The Elective Affinities*. Translated by David Constantine. Oxford World Classics: 2008.

Hillesum, Etty. *An Interrupted Life: The Diaries and Letters from Westerbork 1941–1943*. Picador: 1996.

Hofmannsthal, Hugo von. *Buch der Freunde*. 1922.

Kafka, Franz. *The Zürau Aphorisms*. Translated by Geoffrey Brock and Michael Hofmann. Schocken: 2006.

Kierkegaard, Søren. *The Essential Kierkegaard*. Translated by Howard V. Hong. Princeton University Press: 2000.

Kleist, Heinrich von. *Selected Prose of Heinrich von Kleist*. Translated by Peter Wortsmann. Archipelago: 2009.

Leopardi, Giacomo. *Canti*. Translated by Jonathan Galassi. FSG: 2011.

Leopardi, Giacomo. *Zibaldone*. Translated by Michael Caesar et al. FSG: 2015.

Leopardi, Giacomo. *The Letters of Giacomo Leopardi 1817-1837*. Translated by Prue Shaw. Routledge: 1998.

Marcel, Gabriel. *Homo Viator*. Aubier: 1945.

Minkowski, Eugène. *Lived Time*. Translated by Nancy Wetzel. Northwestern University Press: 2019.

Pascal, Blaise. *Pascal's Thoughts*. Translated by W.F. Trotter. Colliers: 1910.

Pavese, Cesare. *The Business of Living: Diary 1935–1950*. Translated by Geoffrey Brock. Routledge: 2009.

Pavese, Cesare. *Disaffections: Complete Poems 1930-1950*. Translated by Geoffrey Brock. Copper Canyon Press: 2002.

Pavese, Cesare. *Selected Letters 1924-1950*. Translated by A.E. Murch. Peter Owen: 1969.

Péguy, Charles. *Oeuvres poétiques complètes*. Bibliothèque de la Pléiade. Gallimard: 1975.

Pieper, J., Über die Hoffnung, Koesel, München 1949.

Pozzi, A., *Poesia che mi guardi*. G. Bernabò and O. Dino, eds. Sossella: 2010.

Scheler, Max. *Formalism in Ethics and the Non-Formal Ethics of Values*. Translated by Manfred Sings and Roger Funk. Northwestern University Press: 1973.

Trakl, Georg. *Poems and Prose: A Bilingual Edition*. Translated by Alexander Stillmark. Northwestern University Press: 2005.

Weil, Simone. *Waiting for God*. Translated by Emma Crauford. Harper Colophon: 1973.

Weil, Simone. *Intimations of Christianity Among the Ancient Greeks*. Translated by Elisabeth Chase Geissbuhler. Routledge: 1957.

VECTORS

DEFINITION
Vectors are not like typical academic monographs. They are aimed at a more general audience, which might include undergraduate students, academics working in other fields, practitioners, policymakers, and the public. They provide a platform for established academic authors to reach a larger audience than usual, or to speak to new audiences; to deliver bold new arguments; to write unencumbered by the usual obligations for referencing; and to be exciting, provocative and even polemical.

ALREADY PUBLISHED:
Massimo Arcangeli, *Genderless Grammar.*
Alberto Lucarelli, *Tradition & Revolution.*
Eugenio Borgna, *Hope and Despair.*
Eugenio Borgna, *Wounded Nostalgia.*
Eugenio Borgna, *The Madness That is Also in Us.*

COMING SOON:
Simone Gozzano, *Consciousness.*